Lung Embolism

Or, the Scandal of D-Dimer

Constantin Panow

Printed by Createspace

"It is far more important to know what person the disease has, than what disease the person has."

Hippocrates (460-370BC)

4

Disclaimer

The author and publisher decline responsibility about any wrong interpretation or misunderstanding of following text.

Any person in professional practice has highlights or a domain, which he/she particularly affectionate.

Thus, has been for myself the topic of deep venous thrombosis and lung embolism.

As far as I remember, I have tried to do the best out of my knowledge and methods, which were at my disposition.

At first, venous Doppler, more than 30 years ago, then with ultrasound/echography 25 years since, and at last with Angio-scanner of lungs 15-20 years back.

Similar to carrier of any radiologist of my age.

You can't have an idea about this matter, if you are not acquainted with my specialty, and aware about evolution of techniques.

Issue with Doppler

One main problem to be mentioned, is difficulty and learning curve with this modality.

It needs more time to crystallize in your mind, like the perfect one, as it should be!

It attains exquisite quality at turn of century, thanks to computer revolution.

Thus, become visible minute details and thrombi in lower extremities, even less than 1mm in section. (<0.039 inches).

Philosophical Appreciation

As to our daily practice, when I started my training in Radiology, I was already an experienced general practitioner.

In Switzerland at that time we had a different vision about deep venous thrombosis;

(From the one elsewhere, especially USA, as far as I can judge from publications);

And most specialists in internal or general medicine would prescribe anticoagulants in the 80ties, even without 100% proof of disease.

Simply on clinical grounds!

A swollen ankle, with painful leg, in an elderly patient, needed thus no further investigation, but therapy!

I was performing Doppler at that moment, to make sure superficial femoral vein was free.

Only occasionally, we would order phlebography, where this modality was available.

Radiology

Beginning in this profession 1989, I got convinced through personal experience;

And teaching provided to me by an advanced attendee;

About potential of ultrasound for diagnosis of deep venous thrombosis in calf muscles.

Even with machines of this *old time!*

Thus, I started very early in my specialty with this approach.

One such is that most literature coming from USA neglects almost completely ultrasound as a clinical option.

Technicians, instead of physicians, are performing with this tool in the States;

Which is most difficult in Radiology!

Then followed Angio-scanner revolution with spiral and later multi-receptor machines, which provided us with precise depiction of tiny anatomy and very small emboli.

Even better, high resolution images showed so-called *mosaic perfusion* to be the result of chronic variant. (Or longer persistent LE).

Thus, nowadays it is no more mandatory to fix with your eyes for hours small arteries in such an exam, as resorting to much grosser view can give you the right hint.

After diagnosis is established, it becomes easier to obtain second opinion from vessels, which always (or almost) give also the right clue.

Old philosophy

Previous opinions were divergent, but specialists maintained most of the time that this disease is highly lethal.

Most authorities would agree with 20% mortality on every occasion of lung embolism.

Which can be understood only one way:

They meant a massive event in all cases!

News in old fashion

But, as you see, in Mother Nature nothing is mono-valent.

She is profuse in shapes and entities, and arranges herself to put always to shame any scientist.

So-called pulmonary arterial hypertension, which was supposed to be *primary, or so-called essential;*

(Which only means doctors and professors do not know what they are dealing with!)

Was thus vanishing from the scene;

To give place to an old revenant: *Pulmonary embolism!*

Adorned in a garment we did not recognize her before: *A chronic form!*

But who says not acute, implies thus two things:

First, that there is such a stuff like minor thrombi.

Second, that lethality is lesser than in massive entity.

Partiality

Here also lies difficulty of diagnosis, as some authority would not give themselves beaten by arguments alone;

They need also proof of venous thrombi, as well as lung artery emboli.

Modern Ultrasound

To help come modern Doppler machines!

Here, again an issue of learning curve and very long teaching time.

Anatomy

Thorough knowledge of this Specialty in Medicine is mandatory, even more crucial than for Angio-Scan interpretation.

Some radiologists in training are reluctant at learning with this kind of modality, as images are even most difficult to interpret.

But, for whom has started training like myself, first with simple Doppler, then on old Echographs;

Now, doing some Ultrasound with modern technology is nothing but pure pleasure!

Beware

Though, do not forget!

If you do not see thrombi, that does not mean there were none before.

I remember almost observing how a big "*snake*" of 1cm thickness (0.39 inches) moved to the lungs. Within one hour!

And this is even more so of an issue with chronic embolism, where you are searching for a wormling of a few mm (Few times 0.04 inches).

Further Description

Also, if acute and massive disease involves frequently thigh veins, and especially popliteal and superficial femoral vein;

Chronic variety is almost always limited to lower leg. (Calf vessels.)

In 60% to posterior tibial vein;

In 40% concerns fibular ones;

Exclusively anterior tibial is seldom (0.01 %?)

Muscle veins are also participating to a relevant ratio (60-70%).

. Gastrocnemius- most frequently (80%).

. To a lesser degree soleus ones (25-30%).

Physiopathology

We must discuss further about normal mechanisms, which our bodies apply to this disorder.

As we already observed, thrombi have a natural tendency to move to pulmonary bed as emboli.

But why?

Simply because it is only in the lungs, that are present enzymes, able not only to dislodge those amalgams of now foreign material;

(Having no purpose at all!)

But also, and mainly to disperse it and dissolve it;

And at last, bringing it to naught!

Which is the main aim of any organism in its further progression to survival.

Here again, we have differences between those two entities, we are discussing:

If for *acute* and *massive embolism*:

. There is most of the time a precipitating event:

. *"Smoking the pill"*, for instance!

. Or an accident, with lower leg fracture.

. Or hip operation.

Not so for c*hronic variety*:

. Main issue is deficit in Vitamin B 12, which is elevating homocysteine ratio in blood, and thus resulting in a hypercoagulable state.

Here, also belongs our discussion about this parameter.

It is not deep venous thrombosis, which promotes elevation of its amount, but only migration of emboli to the lungs and their dispersion and dissolution!

Also, you understand, that only a lot of material would raise this value above *Normal.*

It is not uncommon to have normal D-Dimer with deep venous thrombosis and lung embolism, even more so with chronic entity.

Doctrine

As to this attitude, you envision after my previous words, that *Lung Embolism* as such is not an *Illness;*

Rather results from natural *Healing Process;*

Or response in our bodies to a hyper-coagulable state.

Only overwhelming factors promote it to a disease condition!

Signs and Symptoms

They are also different, after entity.

Acute one goes with well-known accelerated cardiac rate (Tachycardia), dyspnea, (Tachypnea), and chest pain (Respiratory triggered).

In chronic variety, we have seldom exercise elicited shortness of breath.

(Because disease progresses so slowly, that individuals are unaware of it...)

Labs

Hypoxemia (Hb-desaturation),

Respiratory alkalosis,

S1Q3 on ECG...

Rising D-Dimer.

If for acute variety, only injected CT helps in diagnosis.

(At least, for what most physicians over the Planet think!)

In chronic situation, simple Chest X-Ray is very much contributory!

Remember entity of old!

Known to every doctor as pulmonary arterial hypertension. (PAH)

For which not long ago those guys would propose even Viagra!

Whether this would be helpful in another way?

Now you understand that confirming dilated pulmonary arteries on Chest X-Ray is sufficient to pinpoint diagnosis.

Further, you can substantiate with additional proof, but to my opinion, patients need more treatment of their disease, rather than Radiographical Research.

Anticoagulation!

Chest X-Ray Signs

Of course, all pulmonary arteries are redundant proximally, with a so-called "jump" or acute thinning in their midst.

Here it may be useful to learn lung vessel anatomy on simple pictures.

Tracking those lines, whether they start from right chamber, or end in left entrance.

As their anatomy is a separate, very attractive field on its own.

Reliable Single Warning

But you can attach yourself to *One Original Feature*:

Which is diameter of right pulmonary artery along bronchus intermedius:

Normal: Should not exceed 14 mm (0.55 inches) in women and 16 mm (0.63 inches) in men.

Consequences

Opening of Foramen Ovale:

Seldom in acute embolism.

Almost the rule in chronic cases!

Not so much because flap on this natural opening is *sticky*;

(As it was proposed as explanation for stability of this structure 40 years ago);

Than that it needs time till tricuspid valve becomes incompetent, under progression of PAH;

(Excentric enlargement of right chamber.)

And further raises pressure of right atrium above that of left one.

Complications

Thus, already today's authority confirms 20% of lung embolism cases among brain stroke patients.

Patent foramen ovale is easily seen on cardiac Doppler, and ultrasound;

So, if you are dealing with an elderly person, and symptoms and signs are recent;

Do not doubt!

Just think about this possibility!

Nowadays internists and cardiologists become more aware about this disease;

PFO Once

Which was in no way the case 35 years ago, when I started my carrier.

I remember, that at that time, even making them think about this entity would not help!

No, no anticoagulation!

Well, I was a young physician thence!

Full of enthusiasm and illusions...

Exceptions

There is even a situation, because of which I had always been reluctant prescribing the anti-baby pill to a smoker.

Thrombosis of central retinal artery!

It is said to strike randomly such patients, but with a frequency which had been defined as 0.0001%!

Today I think this was again such a setting, where technology of old time, and applied knowledge, did not allow for correct assignment and concept.

If the subject had been treated differently, simply regular chest X-Ray could have prevented some tragedies.

Turf Battles

One such, is that also peripheral arterial thrombosis, whether of coronary arteries or lower extremities, could be secondary in at least 20% of cases to chronic PE.

But, left heart catheter would not necessarily disclose this disease.

And also, those episodes should not be called thrombotic, but embolic.

Which might be relevant:

If Angiologists (Or Cardiologists) do not see important atherosclerotic changes;

On concerned vessel;

They should question hypothesis of etiology and work to elaborate a better differential.

Therapy

We, medical practitioners, see more and more situations, where a colleague prescribes anticoagulation without end.

Our literature is definite on this topic!

Lung embolism needs treatment for 3-6 months.

Full anticoagulation is mandatory!

Though, what do you do with all those casualties, where there is recurrent disease?

Medical workers become suspicious towards authority, because they do not understand the rationale behind this strategy!

Of course, you have to correct underlying cause of illness, before stopping instituted therapy.

Why not do it right away?

As you can ascertain, that Vitamin B12 deficit is responsible, especially in chronic variety...

Vitamin B12 Shortcoming

This is due to inadequacy of absorption.

As this element is abundant in everyday meals.

It needs for intake through bowel wall so-called Intrinsic Factor;

Secreted by Parietal Cells of stomach.

But in chronic gastritis;

A frequent auto-immune disorder;

We have to deal with paucity of this part in gut lining.

This is how elderly people become deficient in B12 vitamin.

And this to 50% when they are 60 and 80% with 70.

Shortfall Diagnosis

Homocysteine values rise in blood.

Which already by itself is a strong pro-thrombotic factor.

If you feel, as practicing physician, trustworthy to evidence based medicine;

As we all are!

That you need a proof?

Just substitute your patient with Vitamin B12 parenterally.

Don't forget to give also some folic acid by mouth!
As both vitamins work together;

And a long deprivation of first, causes deep lack of second.

Thus, if you do not proceed this way, your patient would need months to stabilize.

Afterwards, you can let his/her homocysteine level be defined again;

And it would confirm no more thrombophilia at all.

At this point, you see, life-long anticoagulation for our elderly population is no more mandatory!

Vitamin substitution instead is sufficient.

No more embarrassment with authority and its confusing decrees!

Statistics

Just, if they say minor elevation of D-Dimer is within normal limits in elderly population...

Tell them again your joke about this matter:

Americans use to say there are three kinds of lies.

(Not only in the States.)

> *– Lies, damned lies, and statistics!*

Personal Experience

I could always demonstrate deep venous thrombosis or lung emboli, or both, in cases of subtly risen D-Dimer.

Differential, of course, is temporary ascent of this value, as for instance in inflammatory illnesses.

Slight LE

Or small one, as a professor of my home-town uttered recently in wide public:

"Who cares?!"

If he would come once to our facility with LE, I should also say *"So, what?!"*

Frequency

This is most difficult subject!

I suspect that most persons, dying all of a sudden, are carried away by LE.

If we try to analyze this topic:

In a big office, having thousands of patients;

There are no more than 3-4 heart infarcts, for which individuals are hospitalized on emergency basis, each year.

So, despite tremendous amount of publications, extensive teaching at medical schools, and continuous reading by trainees in all disciplines;

This is rather a rare disease!

So, why should it be frequent in death?

Cancer, is responsible for 30-40% of casualties in big series.

But, LE can be also secondary to malignancy, as there are so many tumors, which promote a hypercoagulable state.

This percentage is of course difficult to estimate.

But, I pretend, that elderly people would live much longer, on a large scale, if substituted with B12 vitamin.

Pathology

I remember my short training in this specialty.

We were observing those filaments in pulmonary vessels so frequently, that nobody would believe this was LE.

Except Mr Yusuf Kapanci;

(Professor in Chief, Institute Clinical Pathology, Geneva, since 1973-1994);

Lung specialist at that time;

Who would scold us, young practitioners, for having thrown away material from obvious cases.

(Under supervision of elder staff!)

And, what was proposed as first steps of evidence based medicine at that time:

Was proving attachment of those conglomerates to vessel wall.

Nobody would give the fact a thought, that;

If you are looking for such a characteristic;

You should no more call proven events lung emboli;

But rather pulmonary artery thrombosis!

Which, I agree, is extremely rare.

Joke about Plexiform Lesions

Yeah, those guys would even pretend, that such particularities observed on lung biopsy in PAH are no more reversible.

How, the hell, did they know that?

As patients would not survive more than a few years...

And without appropriate therapy, besides!

Confusion

And, on clinical grounds, there has always been a huge turmoil;

Practitioners not being able to understand each other;

Because of the big melting pot of all heart diseases.

Congenital versus acquired ones;

Holding same or similar names, but being completely different entities.

As for instance PFO!

Thus, if you open a book and read about patent foramen ovale;

You would have to take some aspirin after only a few minutes;

Not to keep yours (FO) from closing, of course!

Shunt

So, you said now what kind of a shunt is it?

Right-left or reverse?!

Because with congenital disease you have left-right one (No flap!);

Which continues for a long time without desaturation of hemoglobin;

And direction of blood flow is obvious on heart Doppler...

So, whence the difficulty?

Well, I can only ask!

Here again, those *Specialists* have an *"Explain"*.

They say, because shunt reverses after some years...

Don't tell me!

Systemic circulation;

Which moves the whole body;

And where pressures are 5-10x higher than in lung vessels;

Becomes weaker than pulmonary one?

After both have been trained together;

Why should one get feebler and change direction of blood movement?

Fragility of Physiology

That is, left ventricle, where wall can grow to 5 cm thickness (1.97 inches);

Turns frail and is overrun under pressure of right heart?

Well, perhaps such cases exist!

But their patient is then in a rolling chair, and not walking around, like you and me.

Natural Barrier

Because in between you have the mitral valve;

Which is normal in patent foramen ovale;

And only dilatation of left chamber would ensue in incompetency of it.

But, ventricles react to higher pressures with concentric hypertrophy;

And only much later with enlargement and expansion.

Even better, some colleagues undertake to close those secondary appearing PFO;

With a mechanical device, as if they were handling with inborn Open Ductus Botalli;

And tell the patient, he/she are healed without taking full anticoagulation!

You would say, they prevent access of emboli to systemic circulation.

But, at the expense of worsening pressures in right heart!

Less strokes, but more arrhythmias...

From Scylla to Harybda!

I don't know which one is less lethal.

Chest X-Ray and Frequency Estimate

About 0.2-0.4% of PAH overall. (In Clinics)

In elderly persons, this would be even higher, in vicinity of 0.6-1.5%. (Above 60)

And probably well over 2% in 70 and 5 % in 80 years old ones.

But, of course, bias is that patients come to doctor's office in 50% of conditions for a check-up;

And in another 50% because they feel *"unwell"*.

Here is to mention that we don't know how long it takes till arteries dilate;

And become visible as PAH on chest X-Rays.

Efficiency of Anticoagulation

Vessel diameter reduces rapidly on institution of appropriate treatment.

Long lasting context takes not only prolongated time to diminish artery size, but never returns to "normal" (In my observation).

Thrombophilia diseases

Most severe inherited disorders, like deficit in protein C and S, manifest early in life (In 20-30 years old persons, or even earlier).

Anti-thrombin lll loss is observed in renal disease, especially glomerulonephritis.

Milder forms of pro-thrombotic illnesses can be observed throughout whole lifespan. (Factor V Leiden for instance.)

Survival

I can witness single cases being under observation with chest X-Ray for 3-4 years after PAH was visible. (Without therapy for this disease.)

Gender

PAH and chronic LE is more frequent among women, probably owing to longer natural survival (Than the one of men).

Sensibilisation

Thus, we come to the end of this expose, and my purpose was to make you think a bit about radiological possibilities and our daily routine and practice.

I hope most of you would not take it as a critic, as I am depicting a World-wide disease:

- Not the one of patients,

- But, rather this of doctors!

My goal in this way is to contribute for an incentive on improvement of our strategy concerning this matter, as facts are easy to grasp, within our reach.

I would be glad to exchange views on this subject.

Please, write in my blog!

Website

www.thenopillshealthprospect.com

,